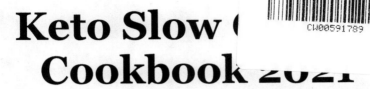

Keto Slow Cooker Cookbook 2021

The Ultimate Amazing and Healthy Recipes to dazzle your Friends.
Mouth-watering, Low-Carb and Tasty Dishes to Lose Weight Fast, Stop Hypertension and Cut Cholesterol.

Melissa Upton

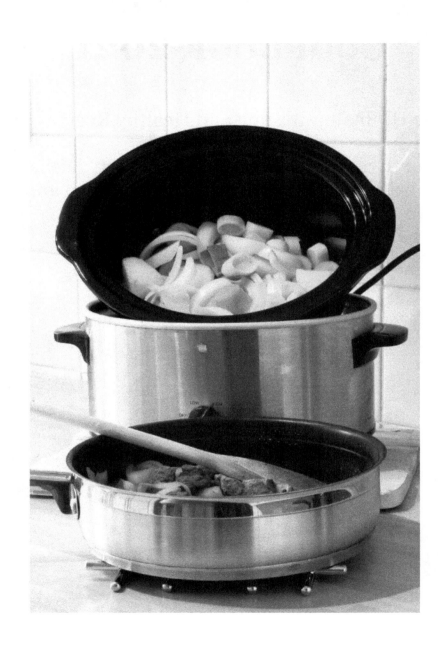

Table of Contents

7

Introduction

Slow cookers can be really useful in the kitchen and can make life so much easier. They make it so that you can prep your ingredients the day before, and they will be ready for you when you get home. The slow cooker is also great for people on a tight budget, because it can save you a lot of money in the long run. That said, it's important to know how to use your slow cooker properly. Here are some tips to help you get started.

Cook With Low Heat

Always start with low heat when cooking your ingredients in a slow cooker. If you put them over medium heat, they will burn or scorch before they are finished. Instead, start out on low heat and let them cook for several hours until they are done. This will ensure that they are safe to eat and don't have any nasty flavors left over from being cooked too fast.

Leave room at the top

Place your ingredients in the cooker as soon as possible after placing them on the stove top or in the oven. This will give them enough time to cook properly without being overcooked on high heat. If you leave them sitting in the hot pot without food inside of it, sometimes it can become stuck and won't release until you turn off the burner. This can cause some parts of your dish to be overcooked, which can ruin everything you worked so hard to perfect!

Use recipes right away

A great way to use your slow cooker is by developing some new recipes! Have fun experimenting and working on some new ones all at once without having to worry about any nasty flavors ruining your dish later on. Take note of what works well and what does not, so you end up with something delicious every time!

Slow Cookers are a great way to prepare your food and make it taste like someone else has done it for you. With the right recipe in your slow cooker, you can turn days of cooking into hours of preparation.

We've decided to share with you some of our favorite slow cooker recipes from around the country. Some recipes are classic favorites, while others are new and fresh. Whatever you're looking for, you'll find it here.

Slow cookers are a great way to prepare all kinds of meals. With the right recipe, you can cook a variety of dishes, including soups that will warm you up on a cold day.

Some of the advantages to using a slow cooker include reducing the amount of energy needed to use your electric stove. You also don't have to worry about burning yourself when using the stove. You can also leave the slow cooker on when you're not home, making it easy to prepare simple meals and snacks for your family.

You can find many recipes in our slow cooker cookbook. It's divided into several sections, including breakfast, main dishes, side dishes, desserts, and drinks. The slow cooker cookbook is designed for a number of different uses. For example, you can use it to make lots of different side dishes and desserts while you're on vacation or traveling. You can also use the same cookbook in your kitchen to prepare healthy main meals during the week or when you're having friends over for dinner.

Don't let your slow cooker get rusty with age! Contact us today to order our slow cooker cookbook at our guaranteed lowest price. We'll even ship it right away so that you can get started cooking immediately!

Vegetable

Vegetable Beef Stew

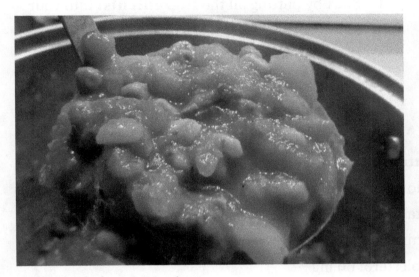

Preparation time: 10 minutes

Cooking time: 8 hours

Servings: 2

Ingredients:

- ½ lb. beef meat, cubed
- ½ yellow onion, diced
- 3 oz. tomato paste
- 1 garlic clove, minced
- ½ tablespoon of thyme, diced
- 1 carrot, diced
- 1.5 celery stalks, diced
- 1 tablespoon of parsley, chopped

- 1 tablespoon of white vinegar
- salt and black pepper to taste

Directions:

1. Start by putting all the **Ingredients:** into your Slow cooker.
2. Cover it and cook for 8 hours on Low settings.
3. Once done, uncover the pot and mix well.
4. Garnish as desired.
5. Serve warm.

Nutrition:

Calories 311

Total Fat 25.5 g

Saturated Fat 12.4 g

Cholesterol 69 mg

Sodium 58 mg

Total Carbs 1.4 g

Fiber 0.7 g

Sugar 7.3 g

Protein 3.4 g

Protein 17.5 g

Spicy Mexican Luncheon

Preparation time: 10 minutes

Cooking time: 8 hours

Servings: 4

Ingredients:

- 2 lbs. beef stew meat, cubed
- 6 tomatoes, diced
- 2 red onion, diced
- 10 oz. canned green chilies, diced
- 4 teaspoon of chili powder
- 2 teaspoon of cumin powder
- 2 teaspoons of oregano, dried
- 4 cups of vegetable broth
- salt and black pepper to taste

Directions:

1. Start by putting all the **Ingredients:** into your Slow cooker.
2. Cover it and cook for 8 hours on Low settings.
3. Once done, uncover the pot and mix well.
4. Garnish as desired.
5. Serve warm.

Nutrition:

Calories 338

Total Fat 34 g

Saturated Fat 8.5 g

Cholesterol 69 mg

Sodium 217 mg

Total Carbs 5.1 g

Fiber 1.2 g

Sugar 12 g

Protein 30.3 g

Beef & Broccoli

Preparation time: 10 minutes

Cooking time: 10 hours

Servings: 4

Ingredients:

- 2 lbs. flank steak, slice into 2" chunks
- 2/3 cup of liquid aminos
- 1 cup of beef broth
- 3 tablespoons of swerve
- 1 teaspoon of freshly grated ginger
- 3 garlic cloves, minced
- 1/4 1/2 teaspoons of red pepper flakes
- 1/2 teaspoons of salt
- 1 head broccoli, diced
- 1 red bell pepper, diced
- 1 teaspoon of sesame seeds

Directions:

1. Start by putting all the **Ingredients:** into your Slow cooker except the broccoli and bell pepper.
2. Cover it and cook for 10 hours on Low settings.
3. Once done, uncover the pot and mix well.
4. Stir in broccoli and bell pepper then continue cooking for 1 hour on low heat.
5. Serve warm.

Nutrition:

Calories 527

Total Fat 49 g

Saturated Fat 14 g

Cholesterol 83 mg

Sodium 92 mg

Total Carbs 3 g

Sugar 1 g

Fiber 1 g

Protein 19 g

Beef Mushroom Stroganoff

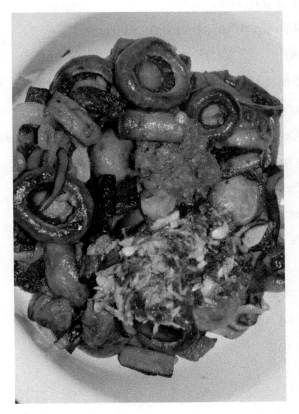

Preparation time: 10 minutes

Cooking time: 8 hours

Servings: 2

Ingredients:

- 1 brown onion sliced and quartered
- 2 cloves garlic, smashed
- 2 slices streaky bacon diced
- 1 lb. beef, stewing steak cubed

- 1 teaspoon of smoked paprika
- 3 tablespoons of tomato paste
- 1 cup of beef stock
- ½ cup of mushrooms quartered

Directions:

1. Start by putting all the Ingredients into your Slow cooker.
2. Cover it and cook for 8 hours on Low settings.
3. Once done, uncover the pot and mix well.
4. Serve warm.

Nutrition:

Calories 416

Total Fat 19.2 g

Saturated Fat 2.4 g

Cholesterol 14 mg

Sodium 261 mg

Total Carbs 3 g

Fiber 2.3 g

Sugar 5.4 g

Protein 41.1 g

Garlic Beef Stew with Olives, Capers, and Tomatoes

Preparation time: 10 minutes

Cooking time: 4 hours

Servings: 6

Ingredients:

- 2 3 lb. beef chuck roast, cut into pieces
- 1 2 tablespoons of olive oil
- 1 can beef broth
- 1 cup of garlic cloves, peeled and cut into lengthwise slivers
- 1 cup of Kalamata Olives, cut in half lengthwise
- 2 tablespoons of capers, rinsed
- 3 bay leaves
- 1 teaspoon of dried Greek oregano
- 1 can (14.5 oz.) tomatoes with juice
- 1 small can (8 oz.) sugar-free tomato sauce
- 2 tablespoons of tomato paste
- 3 tablespoons of red wine vinegar
- fresh black pepper to taste

Directions:

1. Start by putting all the **Ingredients:** into your Slow cooker.
2. Cover it and cook for 4 hours on High settings.

3. Once done, uncover the pot and mix well.

4. Serve warm.

Nutrition:

Calories 378

Total Fat 18.2 g

Saturated Fat 3.1 g

Cholesterol 320 mg

Sodium 130 mg

Total Carbs 2.2 g

Fiber 0.7 g

Sugar 2.7 g

Protein 34.3 g

Mexican Chili

Preparation time: 10 minutes

Cooking time: 8 hours

Servings: 6

Ingredients:

- 2 1/2 lbs. ground beef
- 1 medium red onion, diced and divided
- 4 tablespoons of minced garlic
- 3 large ribs of celery, diced
- ¼ cup of pickled jalapeno slices
- 6 oz. can tomato paste
- 14.5 oz. can tomato and green chilies
- 14.5 oz. can stew tomatoes with Mexican seasoning
- 2 tablespoons of Worcestershire sauce or Coconut Aminos
- 4 tablespoons of chili powder
- 2 tablespoons of cumin, mounded
- 2 teaspoons of salt
- 1/2 teaspoons of cayenne
- 1 teaspoon of garlic powder
- 1 teaspoon of onion powder1 teaspoon of oregano
- 1 teaspoon of black pepper
- 1 bay leaf

Directions:

1. Start by putting all the **Ingredients:** into your Slow cooker.
2. Cover it and cook for 8 hours on Low settings.
3. Once done, uncover the pot and mix well.
4. Serve warm.

Nutrition:

Calories 429

Total Fat 15.1 g

Saturated Fat 9.4 g

Cholesterol 130 mg

Sodium 132 mg

Total Carbs 7 g

Fiber 2.9 g

Sugar 2.4 g

Protein 33.1 g

Green Chile Shredded Beef Cabbage Bowl

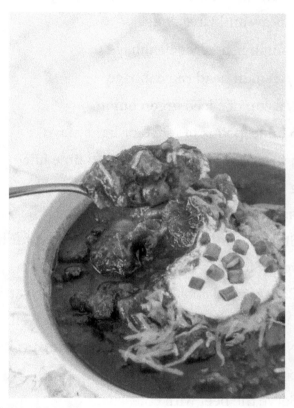

Preparation time: 10 minutes

Cooking time: 4 hours

Servings: 4

Ingredients:

For Slow cooker Beef:

- 2 lb. beef chuck roast, well-trimmed and cut into thick strips
- 1 tablespoon of Kalyn's taco seasoning 2 3 teaspoons of olive oil
- 2 cans (4 oz. can) diced chilis with juice

For Cabbage Slaw and Dressing:

- 1 small head green cabbage
- 1/2 small head red cabbage
- 1/2 cup of sliced green onion
- 6 tablespoons of mayo or light mayo
- 4 teaspoons of fresh-squeezed lime juice
- 2 teaspoons of green Tabasco sauce

Directions:

1. Start by putting all the **Ingredients:** for beef into your Slow cooker.
2. Cover it and cook for 4 hours on High settings.
3. Once done, uncover the pot and mix well.
4. Now toss all the coleslaw **Ingredients:** in a salad bowl.
5. Serve the beef with coleslaw.

Nutrition:

Calories 429

Total Fat 11.9 g

Saturated Fat 1.7 g

Cholesterol 78 mg

Sodium 79 mg

Total Carbs 1.8 g

Fiber 1.1 g

Sugar 0.3 g

Protein 35 g

Chipotle Barbacoa Recipe

Preparation time: 10 minutes

Cooking time: 10 hours

Servings: 6

Ingredients:

- 3 lb. beef brisket or chuck roast
- 1/2 cup of beef broth
- 2 medium chipotle chilis in adobo
- 5 cloves garlic
- 2 tablespoons of apple cider vinegar
- 2 tablespoons of lime juice
- 1 tablespoon of oregano, dried
- 2 teaspoons of cumin
- 2 teaspoons of salt
- 1 teaspoon of black pepper
- 1/2 teaspoons of cloves, ground
- 2 whole bay leaf

Directions:

1. Start by putting all the **Ingredients:** into your Slow cooker.
2. Cover it and cook for 10 hours on Low settings.
3. Once done, uncover the pot and mix well.
4. Shred the slow-cooked beef and return it to the pot.
5. Serve warm.

Nutrition:

Calories 248

Total Fat 15.7 g

Saturated Fat 2.7 g

Cholesterol 75 mg

Sodium 94 mg

Total Carbs 4.4 g

Fiber 0.2 g

Sugar 0.1 g

Protein 43.2 g

Beef Dip

Preparation time: 10 minutes

Cooking time: 10 hours

Servings: 6

Ingredients

- ½ cup heavy cream

- 1 onion, diced

- 1 teaspoon cream cheese

- ½ cup Cheddar cheese, shredded

- 1 teaspoon garlic powder

- oz. dried beef, chopped

- ½ cup of water

Directions

1   Put all **Ingredients:** in the slow cooker.

2   Gently stir the **Ingredients:** and close the lid.

3   Cook the dip on Low for 10 hours.

Nutrition:

118 calories,

8.6g protein,

2.5g carbohydrates,

8.2g fat,

0.4g fiber,

41mg cholesterol,

78mg sodium,

126mg potassium.

Beef and Sauerkraut Bowl

Preparation time: 10 minutes

Cooking time: 5 hours

Servings: 4

Ingredients

- 1 cup sauerkraut

- 1-pound corned beef, chopped

- ¼ cup apple cider vinegar

- 1 cup of water

Directions

1   Pour water and apple cider vinegar into the slow cooker.

2   Add corned beef and cook it on High for 5 hours.

3   Then chop the meat roughly and put in the serving bowls.

4   Top the meat with sauerkraut.

Nutrition:

202 calories,

15.5g protein,

1.7g carbohydrates,

14.2g fat,

1g fiber,

71mg cholesterol,

1240mg sodium,

236mg potassium

Sweet Passata Dipped Steaks

Preparation time: 10 minutes

Cooking time: 2 hours

Servings: 4

Ingredients:

- ¼ cup of Tomato passata
- 1 teaspoon of Ginger, grated
- 1 tablespoon of Mustard
- 1 Garlic clove, minced
- 1 teaspoon of Garlic, minced
- 1 tablespoon of Stevia
- 1 tablespoon of Olive oil
- 1 and ½ lbs. Beef steaks

Directions:

1. Start by putting all the **Ingredients:** into your Slow cooker.
2. Cover it and cook for 2 hours on High settings.
3. Once done, uncover the pot and mix well.
4. Garnish as desired.
5. Serve warm.

Nutrition:

Calories 371

Total Fat 17.2 g

Saturated Fat 9.4 g

Cholesterol 141 mg

Sodium 153 mg

Total Carbs 6 g

Fiber 0.9 g

Sugar 1.4 g

Protein 32 g

Mushroom Beef Goulash

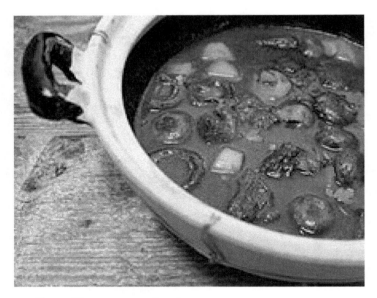

Preparation time: 10 minutes

Cooking time: 8 hours

Servings: 3

Ingredients:

- 1 and ½ lbs. beef, cubed
- 1 red bell pepper, diced
- 1 yellow onion, diced
- 2 garlic cloves, minced
- 2 teaspoons of sweet paprika
- 3 oz. mushrooms halved
- 2 bay leaves
- a drizzle of olive oil
- ½ cup of beef stock

- ½ cup of coconut cream

Directions:

1. Start by putting all the **Ingredients:** into your Slow cooker.
2. Cover it and cook for 8 hours on Low settings.
3. Once done, uncover the pot and mix well.
4. Remove and discard the bay leaves.
5. Garnish as desired.
6. Serve warm.

Nutrition:

Calories 291

Total Fat 14.2 g

Saturated Fat 4.4 g

Cholesterol 180 mg

Sodium 154 mg

Total Carbs 5.3 g

Fiber 3.1 g

Sugar 3.6 g

Protein 20.8 g

Beef Onion Stew

Preparation time: 10 minutes

Cooking time: 4 hours

Servings: 2

Ingredients:

- 1 tablespoon of olive oil
- 1 yellow onion, diced
- 1 lb. beefsteak, cut into strips
- 2 springs onions, diced
- 1 cup of tomato passata
- Salt and black pepper- to taste

Directions:

1. Start by putting all the **Ingredients:** into your Slow cooker except the spring onions.
2. Cover it and cook for 4 hours on medium settings.
3. Once done, uncover the pot and mix well.
4. Garnish with spring onions.
5. Serve warm.

Nutrition:

Calories 419

Total Fat 13.2 g

Saturated Fat 21.4 g

Cholesterol 140 mg

Sodium 161 mg

Total Carbs 3.5 g

Fiber 2.9 g

Sugar 3.4 g

Protein 36.2 g

Beef Steaks with Peppercorn Sauce

Preparation time: 10 minutes

Cooking time: 8 hours

Servings: 2

Ingredients:

- 2 medium sirloin beef steaks
- 1 teaspoon of black peppercorns
- ¼ cup of sugar-free tomato sauce
- Salt and black pepper- to taste
- 1 tablespoon of olive oil

Directions:

1. Start by putting all the **Ingredients:** into your Slow cooker.
2. Cover it and cook for 8 hours on Low settings.
3. Once done, uncover the pot and mix well.
4. Garnish as desired.
5. Serve warm.

Nutrition:

Calories 351

Total Fat 12.2 g

Saturated Fat 2.4 g

Cholesterol 110 mg

Sodium 276 mg

Total Carbs 5.4 g

Fiber 0.9 g

Sugar 1.4 g

Protein 15.8 g

Pumpkin Beef Chili

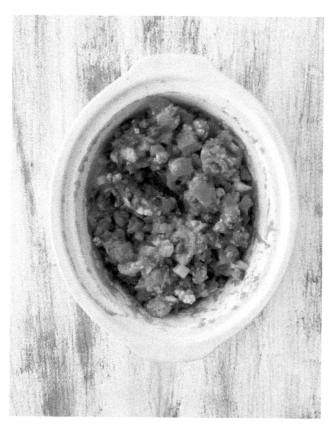

Preparation time: 10 minutes

Cooking time: 3 hours

Servings: 6

Ingredients:

- 1 tablespoon of Olive oil
- 1 green bell pepper, diced
- 1 ½ lb. Beef, ground
- 6 garlic cloves, minced

- 28 oz. canned tomatoes, diced
- 14 oz. pumpkin puree
- 1 cup of chicken stock
- 2 tablespoon of Chili powder
- 1 ½ teaspoon of Cumin, ground
- 1 teaspoon of Cinnamon powder
- Salt and black pepper- to taste

Directions:

1. Start by putting all the **Ingredients:** into your Slow cooker.
2. Cover it and cook for 4 hours on Low settings.
3. Once done, uncover the pot and mix well.
4. Garnish as desired.
5. Serve warm.

Nutrition:

Calories 238

Total Fat 13.8 g

Saturated Fat 1.7 g

Cholesterol 221 mg

Sodium 120 mg

Total Carbs 4.3 g

Fiber 2.4 g

Sugar 11.2 g

Protein 34.4g

Olives Beef Stew

Preparation time: 10 minutes

Cooking time: 10 hours

Servings: 4

Ingredients:

- 28 oz. beefsteak, cubed
- 1 tablespoon of olive oil
- 1 tablespoon of parsley, chopped
- Salt and black pepper- to taste
- 8 oz. tomato passata
- 1 yellow onion, diced
- 1 cup of green olives pitted and sliced

Directions:

1. Start by putting all the **Ingredients:** into your Slow cooker.
2. Cover it and cook for 10 hours on Low settings.
3. Once done, uncover the pot and mix well.
4. Garnish as desired.
5. Serve warm.

Nutrition:

Calories 359

Total Fat 34 g

Saturated Fat 10.3 g

Cholesterol 112 mg

Total Carbs 8.5 g

Sugar 2 g

Fiber 1.3 g

Sodium 92 mg

Protein 27.5 g

Pulled Pork

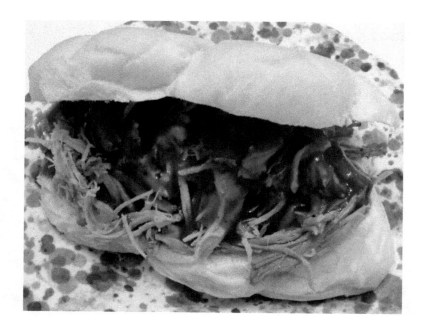

Preparation time: 5 minutes

Cooking time: 8 hours

Servings: 8

Ingredients

- 3 pounds pasture-raised pork shoulder, boneless and fat trimmed

- 2 teaspoons onion powder

- 2 teaspoons garlic powder

- 2 teaspoons salt

- 2 teaspoons paprika

- 1 tablespoon parsley

- 2 teaspoons cumin

- ½ cup beer

Directions:

1. Place pork in a 6-quart slow cooker and switch it on.

2. Stir together remaining **Ingredients:** except for beer and then rub this mixture all over the pork until evenly coated on all sides.

3. Pour in beer, then shut with lid and cook for 8 hours at low heating setting or 4 hours at high heat setting.

4. When done, shred pork with two forks; stir well until coated with sauce and serve.

Nutrition: Net Carbs: 2g; Calories: 233; Total Fat: 12g; Saturated Fat: 3g; Protein: 20g; Carbs: 2g; Fiber: 0g; Sugar: 0g

Pork Roast

Preparation time: 5 minutes

Cooking time: 8 hours and 15 minutes

Servings: 6

Ingredients

- 30-ounce pasture-raised pork shoulder, fat trimmed

- 1 teaspoon minced garlic

- ½ teaspoon grated ginger

- ½ tablespoon salt

- ½ teaspoon ground black pepper

- 2 teaspoons dried thyme

- 1 tablespoon paprika powder

- 5 black peppercorns

- 1 bay leaf

- 1 tablespoon avocado oil

- 1 cup water

Directions:

1. Place pork in a 6-quart slow cooker, season with salt and thyme, add peppercorns and bay leaf and then pour in water.

---

2. Plug in the slow cooker, then shut with its lid and cook for 8 hours at low heat setting or 4 hours at high heat setting.

3. When done, transfer pork to a baking dish and reserve cooking sauce in a saucepan.

4. Set oven to 450 degrees F and let preheat.

5. In the meantime, stir together remaining **Ingredients:** in a small bowl until combined and then brush mixture all over pork.

6. Place the baking sheet into the oven to bake pork for 10 to 15 minutes or until roasted.

7. Cut roasted pork into thin slices and serve with reserved cooking sauce.

Nutrition: Net Carbs: 3g; Calories: 579; Total Fat: 51g; Saturated Fat: 12g; Protein: 28g; Carbs: 4g; Fiber: 1g; Sugar: 0.1g

Chinese Pulled Pork

Preparation time: 5 minutes

Cooking time: 7 hours and 30 minutes

Servings: 6

Ingredients

- 2.2-pound pasture-raised pork shoulder, fat trimmed

- 2 tablespoons garlic paste

- 2 teaspoons ginger paste

- 1 teaspoon smoked paprika

- 5 drops Erythritol sweetener

- 4 tablespoons soy sauce

- 1 tablespoon tomato paste

- 4 tablespoons tomato sauce, sugar-free

- 1 cup chicken broth

Directions:

1. Place pork in a 6-quart slow cooker.

2. Whisk together remaining **Ingredients:** until smooth and then pour over the pork.

3. Plug in the slow cooker, then shut with lid and cook for 7 hours at low heat setting or until pork is tender.

---

4. Then shred pork with two forks and stir well until evenly coated with sauce.

5. Continue cooking pork for 30 minutes or more at low heating setting until sauce is thicken to desired consistency.

6. Serve straightaway.

Nutrition: Net Carbs: 2g; Calories: 447; Total Fat: 35g; Saturated Fat: 13g; Protein: 30g; Carbs: 3g; Fiber: 1g; Sugar: 2g

Bacon Wrapped Pork Loin

Preparation time: 5 minutes

Cooking time: 7 hours

Servings: 4

Ingredients

- 2-pound pasture-raised pork loin roast, fat-trimmed

- 4 strips of bacon, uncooked

- 3 tablespoon dried onion soup mix, organic

- 1/4 cup water

Directions:

1. Pour water into a 6-quart slow cooker.

2. Rub seasoning mix on all sides of pork, then wrap with bacon and place into the slow cooker.

3. Plug in the slow cooker, then shut with lid and cook for seven hours at low heat setting or 5 hours at high heat setting.

4. Serve straightaway.

Nutrition: Net Carbs: 0g; Calories: 639; Total Fat: 41g; Saturated Fat: 19g; Protein: 69g; Carbs: 0g; Fiber: 0g; Sugar: 0g

Lasagna

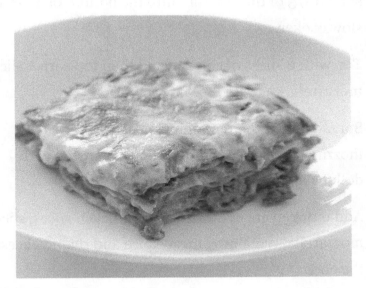

Preparation time: 10 minutes

Cooking time: 3 hours

Servings: 8

Ingredients

- 2 pounds minced pasture-raised pork, browned and fat drained

- 16 slices of chicken thin deli slices

- 24-ounce marinara sauce, organic and sugar-free

- 15-ounce ricotta cheese

- 12 slices of mozzarella cheese

- 1 ½ cups shredded mozzarella cheese

Directions:

1. Stir together pork and marinara sauce in a bowl and spread 1/3 of this mixture into the bottom of a 6-quarts slow cooker.

2. Top with 8 slices of chicken and then top with 6 slices of mozzarella cheese.

3. Spread half of the remaining meat mixture over mozzarella cheese layer and then evenly top with dollops of half of the ricotta cheese.

4. Add more layers by starting with chicken slices, slices of mozzarella, remaining meat sauce and ricotta cheese in the end.

5. Top with shredded mozzarella cheese, then plug in the slow cooker, shut with lid and cook for 2 to 3 hours at low heat setting or until cheeses melt completely.

6. When done, let the slow cooker cool for 1 hour and then slice lasagna and serve immediately.

Nutrition: Net Carbs: 6g; Calories: 720; Total Fat: 53g; Saturated Fat: 17g; Protein: 50g; Carbs: 11g; Fiber: 5g; Sugar: 5g

Meatballs Stuffed With Cheese

Preparation time: 5 minutes

Cooking time: 6 hours

Servings: 4

Ingredients

- 2 1/2 pounds ground pork, pasture-raised

- 1/2 cup pork rinds, crushed

- 1/2 teaspoon garlic powder

- 1/2 teaspoon salt

- 1/2 teaspoon ground black pepper

- 2 tablespoons Italian seasonings

- 2 cup marinara sauce, sugar-free and organic

- 2 eggs

- 1/2 cup grated Parmesan cheese

- 8 ounces block of mozzarella cheese, cut into 24 pieces

Directions:

1. Crack eggs in a large bowl, add pork rind, garlic powder, salt, black pepper, and Italian seasoning and whisk until combined.

2. Add ground meat, then mix until combined and shape the mixture into 24 meatballs.

3. Place a piece of cheese into the center of each meatball and then wrap meat around it.

4. Pour half of the marinara sauce into the bottom of a 6-quart slow cooker, then arrange meatballs and cover with remaining sauce.

5. Plug in the slow cooker, shut with lid and cook meatballs for 6 hours at low heat setting or 3 hours at high heat setting.

6. Serve straightaway.

Nutrition: Net Carbs: 6.5g; Calories: 548; Total Fat: 34g; Saturated Fat: 10g; Protein: 49g; Carbs: 9.5g; Fiber: 3g; Sugar: 4g

Kalua Pig

Preparation time: 5 minutes
Cooking time: 16 hours
Servings: 8
Ingredients

- 5 pounds pasture-raised pork shoulder, bone-in, and fat-trimmed

- 3 slices of bacon

- 5 cloves of garlic, peeled

- 2 tablespoons sea salt

Directions:

1. Make some cuts into the pork, then tuck garlic in them and season with salt.

2. Line a 6-quarts slow cooker with bacon slices, then top with seasoned pork and shut with lid.

3. Plug in the slow cooker and cook for 16 hours at low heat setting until very tender.

4. When done, transfer pork to a cutting board and shred pork with two forks.

5. Then taste pork to adjust seasoning and add cooking liquid to adjust seasoning.

6. Serve straightaway.

Nutrition: Net Carbs: 0g; Calories: 349; Total Fat: 27g; Saturated Fat: 10g; Protein: 26.6g; Carbs: 0g; Fiber: 0g; Sugar: 0g

Balsamic Pork Tenderloin

Preparation time: 5 minutes

Cooking time: 6 hours

 Servings: 8

Ingredients

- 2 pounds pasture-raised pork tenderloin

- 2 teaspoons minced garlic

- 1/2 teaspoon sea salt

- 1/2 teaspoon red pepper flakes

- 1 tablespoon Worcestershire sauce

- 2 tablespoons avocado oil

- 1/2 cup balsamic vinegar

- 2 tablespoons coconut aminos

Directions:

1. Grease a 6-quart slow cooker with oil and set aside.

2. Sprinkle garlic all over the pork and then place it into the slow cooker.

3. Whisk together remaining Ingredients, then pour over pork and shut with lid.

4. Plug in the slow cooker and cook pork for 6 hours at low heat setting or 4 hours at high setting until tender.

---

5. When done, transfer pork to serving plate, pour ½ cup of cooking liquid over pork and serve.

Nutrition: Net Carbs: 0.6g; Calories: 224; Total Fat: 10g; Saturated Fat: 1.6g; Protein: 33g; Carbs: 0.6g; Fiber: 0g; Sugar: 0.3g

Spicy Pork

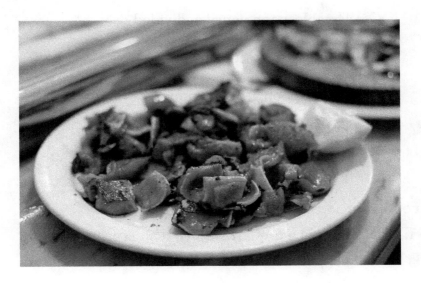

Preparation time: 5 minutes

Cooking time: 10 hours

Servings: 6

Ingredients

- 2 pasture-raised pork shoulder, boneless and fat trimmed

- ½ of jalapeno, deseeded and cored, chopped

- 6 ounce crushed tomatoes

- ¼ cup chopped green onion

- 3 clove of garlic, peeled and sliced in half

- 1 tablespoon sea salt

- ½ teaspoon ground black pepper

- 1 ½ tablespoon paprika, divided

- ½ tablespoon dried oregano

- ½ tablespoon ground cumin

- 2 limes, juiced

- 2 tablespoons avocado oil

Directions:

1. Place pork in a 6-quart slow cooker, season with salt, black pepper, paprika, oregano, and cumin until seasoned well.

2. Then add remaining Ingredients and stir until combined.

3. Plug in the slow cooker, shut it with the lid and cook for 8 to 10 hours at low heat setting or 4 to 5 hours at high heat setting until very tender.

4. Serve straightaway.

Nutrition: Net Carbs: 1.2g; Calories: 344.5; Total Fat: 25g; Saturated Fat: 10.7g; Protein: 28.4g; Carbs: 1.7g; Fiber: 0.5g; Sugar: 1.1g

Zesty Garlic Pulled Pork

Preparation time: 5 minutes

Cooking time: 8 hours

Servings: 6

Ingredients

- 3-pound pasture-raised pork shoulder

- 5 cloves of garlic, peeled and sliced

- 1 tablespoon of salt

- 1/2 teaspoon ground black pepper

- 1 teaspoon oregano

- 1/2 teaspoon cumin

- 1 lime, zested and juiced

Directions:

1. Make cut into the meat of pork and stuff with garlic slices.

2. Stir together garlic, salt, black pepper, oregano, cumin, lime zest, and juice until smooth paste comes together and then brush this paste all over the pork.

3. Place pork into a large resealable bag, seal it and let marinate in the refrigerator for overnight.

4. When ready to cook, transfer pork to a 6-quart slow cooker and shut with lid.

5. Plug in the slow cooker and cook for 8 hours at low heat setting or until pork is very tender.

6. When done, shred pork with two forks and serve as a lettuce wrap.

Nutrition: Net Carbs: 1.2g; Calories: 616; Total Fat: 43g; Saturated Fat: 11.5g; Protein: 55.4g; Carbs: 1.5g; Fiber: 0.3g; Sugar: 0g

Ranch Pork Chops

Preparation time: 5 minutes

Cooking time: 8 hours

Servings: 6

Ingredients

- 8-ounce sliced mushrooms

- 2 pounds pasture-raised pork loin

- 2 tablespoons ranch dressing mix

- 2 tablespoons avocado oil

- 21 ounce cream of chicken soup

- 2 cups water

Directions:

1. Add ranch dressing, oil chicken soup, and water into the bowl, whisk until smooth, then add mushrooms and stir until combined.

2. Cut pork into 6 slices and layer into the bottom of a slow cooker.

3. Evenly pour in prepared chicken soup mixture and shut with lid.

4. Plug in the slow cooker and cook for eight hours at low heat setting or until pork is cooked through.

5. Serve straightaway.

Nutrition: Net Carbs: 4g; Calories: 479; Total Fat: 27g; Saturated Fat: 12g; Protein: 54g; Carbs: 5g; Fiber: 1g; Sugar: 1.5g

Clam Chowder

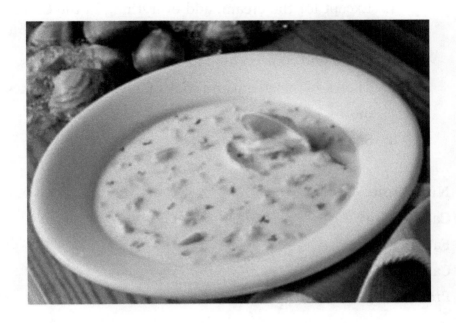

Preparation time: 10 minutes

Cooking time: 2 hours

Servings: 4

Ingredients:

- Chopped celery – ½ cup
- Chopped onion – ½ cup
- Chicken broth – 1 cup
- Whole baby clams with juice – 2 cans
- Heavy whipping cream – 1 cup
- Salt – ½ tsp.
- Ground thyme – ½ tsp.

- Pepper – ½ tsp.

Directions:

1. Except for the cream, add everything in the Crock-Pot.
2. Cover and cook on high for 1 hour and 45 minutes.
3. Then add the cream and cook on high for 15 minutes more.
4. Serve.

Nutrition:

Calories: 427

Fat: 33g

Carbs: 5g

Protein: 27g

Creamy Seafood Chowder

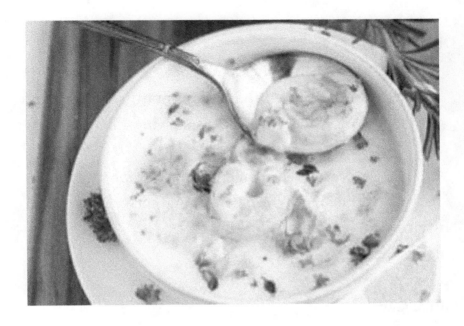

Preparation time: 10 minutes

Cooking time: 5 hours

Servings: 6

Ingredients:

- Garlic – 5 cloves, crushed
- Small onion – 1, finely chopped
- Prawns – 1 cup
- Shrimp – 1 cup
- Whitefish – 1 cup
- Full-fat cream – 2 cups
- Dry white wine – 1 cup

- A handful of fresh parsley, finely chopped
- Olive oil – 2 tbsp.

Directions:

1. Drizzle oil into the Crock-Pot.
2. Add the white fish, shrimp, prawns, onion, garlic, cream, wine, salt, and pepper into the pot. Stir to mix.
3. Cover with the lid and cook on low for 5 hours.
4. Sprinkle with fresh parsley and serve.

Nutrition:

Calories: 225

Fat: 9.6g

Carbs: 5.6g

Protein: 21.4g

Salmon Cake

Preparation time: 10 minutes

Cooking time: 4 hours

Servings: 4

Ingredients:

- Eggs – 4, lightly beaten
- Heavy cream – 3 tbsp.
- Baby spinach – 1 cup, roughly chopped
- Smoked salmon strips – 4 ounces, chopped
- A handful of fresh coriander, roughly chopped
- Olive oil – 2 tbsp.
- Salt and pepper to taste

Directions:

1. Drizzle oil into the Crock-Pot.
2. Place the spinach, cream, beaten egg, salmon, salt, and pepper into the pot and mix to combine.
3. Cover with the lid and cook on low for 4 hours.

Nutrition:

Calories: 277

Fat: 20.8g

Carbs: 1.1g

Protein: 22.5g

Lemon-Butter Fish

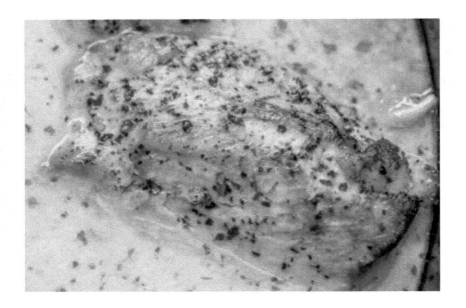

Preparation time: 10 minutes

Cooking time: 5 hours

Servings: 4

Ingredients:

- Fresh white fish – 4 fillets
- Butter - 1 ½ ounce, soft but not melted
- Garlic cloves – 2, crushed
- Lemon – 1 (juice and zest)
- A handful of fresh parsley, finely chopped
- Salt and pepper to taste
- Olive oil – 2 tbsp.

Directions:

1. Combine the butter, garlic, zest of one lemon, and chopped parsley to a bowl.
2. Drizzle oil into the Crock-Pot.
3. Season the fish with salt and pepper and place into the pot.
4. Place a dollop of lemon butter onto each fish fillet and gently spread it out.
5. Cover with the lid and cook on low for 5 hours.
6. Serve each fish fillet with a generous spoonful of melted lemon butter from the bottom of the pot. Drizzle with lemon juice and serve.

Nutrition:

Calories: 202

Fat: 13.4g

Carbs: 1.3g

Protein: 20.3g

Salmon with Green Beans

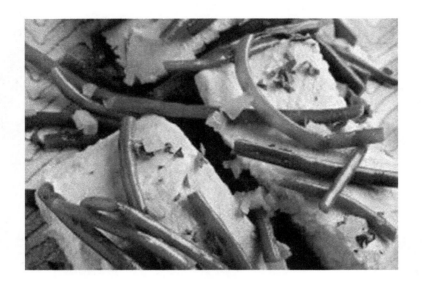

Preparation time: 10 minutes

Cooking time: 3 hours

Servings: 4

Ingredients:

- Salmon fillets – 4, skin on
- Garlic – 4 cloves, crushed
- Broccoli – ½ head, cut into florets
- Frozen green beans – 2 cups
- Olive oil – 3 tbsp., divided
- Salt and pepper to taste
- Water – ¼ cup

Directions:

1. Add the olive oil into the Crock-Pot.
2. Season the salmon with salt and pepper and place into the pot (skin-side down). Add the water.
3. Place garlic, beans, and broccoli on top of the salmon. Season with salt and pepper.
4. Drizzle some more oil over the veggies and fish.
5. Cover with the lid and cook on high for 3 hours.
6. Serve.

Nutrition:

Calories: 278

Fat: 17.8g

Carbs: 8.1g

Protein: 24.5g

Coconut Fish Curry

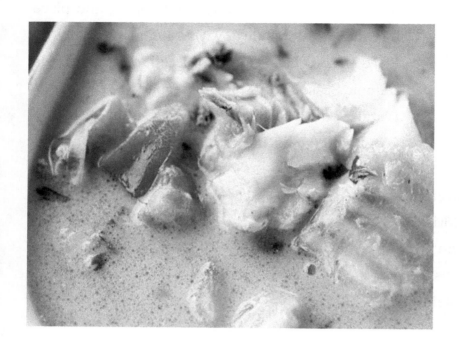

Preparation time: 10 minutes

Cooking time: 4 hours

Servings: 4

Ingredients:

- Large white fish fillets – 4, cut into chunks
- Garlic cloves – 4, crushed
- Small onion – 1, finely chopped
- Ground turmeric – 1 tsp.
- Yellow curry paste – 2 tbsp.
- Fish stock – 2 cups

- Full-fat coconut milk – 2 cans
- Lime – 1
- Fresh coriander as needed, roughly chopped
- Olive oil – 2 tbsp.
- Salt and pepper to taste

Directions:

1. Add olive oil into the Crock-Pot.
2. Add the coconut milk, stock, fish, curry paste, turmeric, onion, garlic, salt, and pepper to the pot. Stir to combine.
3. Cover with the lid and cook on high for 4 hours.
4. Drizzle with lime juice and fresh coriander and serve.

Nutrition:

Calories: 562

Fat: 49.9g

Carbs: 13g

Protein: 20.6g

Coconut Lime Mussels

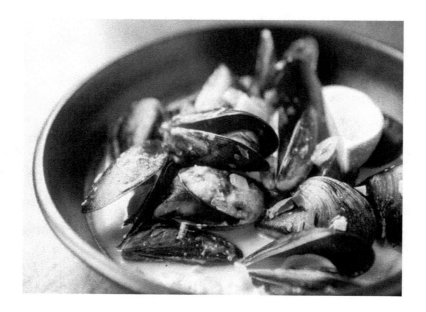

Preparation time: 10 minutes

Cooking time: 2 ½ hours

Servings: 4

Ingredients:

- Fresh mussels – 16
- Garlic – 4 cloves
- Full-fat coconut milk – 1 ½ cups
- Red chili – ½, finely chopped
- Lime – 1, juiced
- Fish stock – ½ cup
- A handful of fresh coriander

- Olive oil – 2 tbsp.
- Salt and pepper to taste

Directions:

1. Add olive oil into the Crock-Pot.
2. Add the coconut milk, garlic, chili, fish stock, salt, pepper, and juice of one lime to the pot. Stir to mix.
3. Cover with the lid and cook on high for 2 hours.
4. Remove the lid, place mussels into the liquid, and cover with the lid.
5. Cook until mussels open, about 20 minutes.
6. Serve the mussels with pot sauce. Garnish with fresh coriander.

Nutrition:

Calories: 342

Fat: 30.2g

Carbs: 11.3g

Protein: 10.9g

Calamari, Prawn, and Shrimp Pasta Sauce

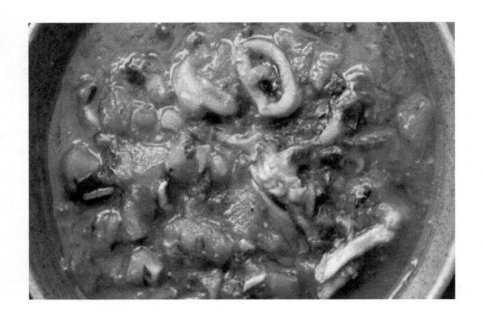

Preparation time: 10 minutes

Cooking time: 3 hours

Servings: 4

Ingredients:

- Calamari – 1 cup

- Prawns – 1 cup
- Shrimp – 1 cup
- Garlic – 6 cloves, crushed
- Tomatoes – 4, chopped
- Dried mixed herbs – 1 tsp.

- Balsamic vinegar - 1 tbsp.
- Olive oil – 2 tbsp.
- Salt and pepper to taste
- Water – ½ cup

Directions:

1. Add oil into the Crock-Pot.
2. Add the tomatoes, garlic, shrimp, prawns, calamari, mixed herbs, balsamic vinegar, water, salt, and pepper. Stir to mix.
3. Cover with the lid and cook on high for 3 hours.
4. Serve with zucchini noodles or veggies.

Nutrition:

- Calories: 372
- Fat: 14.6g
- Carbs: 8.5g
- Protein: 55.1g

Sesame Prawns

Preparation time: 10 minutes

Cooking time: 2 hours

Servings: 4

Ingredients:

- Large prawns – 3 cups
- Garlic – 4 cloves, crushed
- Sesame oil – 1 tbsp.
- Toasted sesame seeds – 2 tbsp.
- Red chili – ½, finely chopped
- Fish stock – ½ cup
- Salt and pepper to taste
- Chopped herbs for serving

Directions:

1. Drizzle the sesame oil into the Crock-Pot.
2. Add the garlic, prawns, sesame seeds, chili, and fish stock to the pot. Mix to coat.
3. Cover with the lid and cook on high for 2 hours.
4. Serve hot with fresh herbs and cauliflower rice.

Nutrition:

- Calories: 236
- Fat: 7.7g
- Carbs: 4.3g
- Protein: 37.4g

Tuna Steaks

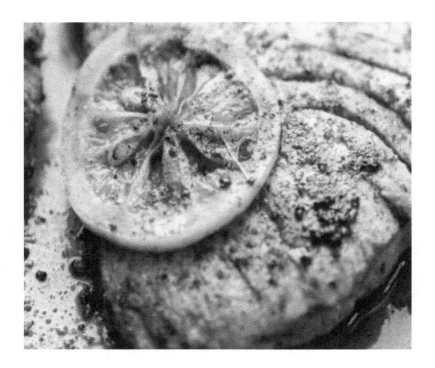

Preparation time: 10 minutes

Cooking time: 3 hours

Servings: 4

Ingredients:

- Tuna steaks – 4
- Garlic – 3 cloves, crushed
- Lemon – 1, sliced into 8 slices
- White wine – ½ cup
- Olive oil – 2 tbsp.
- Salt and pepper to taste

Directions:

1. Reduce the white wine in a pan by simmering until the strong alcohol smell is cooked off.
2. Rub the tuna steaks with olive oil, and season with salt and pepper.
3. Place the tuna steaks into the Crock-Pot.
4. Sprinkle the crushed garlic on top of the tuna steaks.
5. Place 2 lemon slices on top of each tuna steak.
6. Pour the reduced wine into the pot.
7. Cover with the lid and cook on high for 3 hours.
8. Transfer fish on serving plates. Drizzle with pot liquid and serve.

Nutrition:

Calories: 269

Fat: 8.6g

Carbs: 2.9g

Protein: 40.4g

Creamy Smoked Salmon Soup

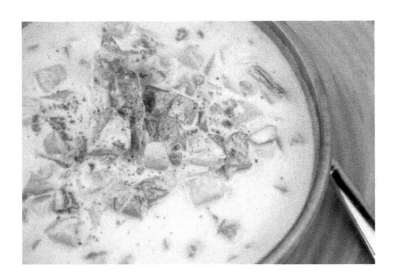

Preparation time: 10 minutes

Cooking time: 3 hours

Servings: 4

Ingredients:

- Smoked salmon – ½ lb., roughly chopped
- Garlic – 3 cloves, crushed
- Small onion – 1, finely chopped
- Leek – 1, finely chopped
- Heavy cream – 1 ½ cups
- Olive oil – 2 tbsp.
- Salt and pepper to taste

- Fish stock – 1 ½ cups

Directions:

1. Add oil into the Crock-Pot.
2. Add fish stock, leek, salmon, garlic, and onion into the pot.
3. Cover with the lid and cook on low for 2 hours.
4. Add the cream and stir. Cook for 1 hour more.
5. Adjust seasoning and serve.

Nutrition:

Calories: 309

Fat: 26.4g

Carbs: 7g

Protein: 12.3g

Cheese and Prawns

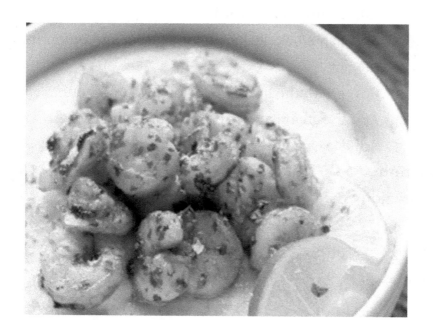

Preparation time: 10 minutes

Cooking time: 1 hour 20 minutes

Servings: 4

Ingredients:

- Shallots – 2, finely chopped
- Apple cider vinegar – ¼ cup
- Butter – 2 tbsp.
- Raw prawns – 4 lbs., peeled, rinsed, patted dry
- Almond meal – 2 tsp.
- Swiss cheese – 1 cup, grated
- Garlic – 2 cloves, peeled, thinly sliced

- Hot pepper sauce – ¼ tsp.
- Salt to taste
- Fresh parsley to serve

Directions:

1. Melt butter in a skillet over medium heat. Then add shallots and sauté for a few minutes until translucent.
2. Add prawns and sauté for 2 minutes. Set aside.
3. Grease the inside of the pot with a little butter.
4. Sprinkle garlic over it and add cheese.
5. In a bowl, mix almond meal, apple cider, and hot sauce. Pour the mixture into the Crock-Pot. Stir.
6. Cover and cook on low for 1 hour.
7. Add the prawn shallot mixture and stir.
8. Cover and cook on low for 10 minutes.
9. Stir again and sprinkle parsley over it.
10. Serve.

Nutrition:

Calories: 238

Fat: 13.5g

Carbs: 9g

Protein: 20g

Cheesy Salmon Bites

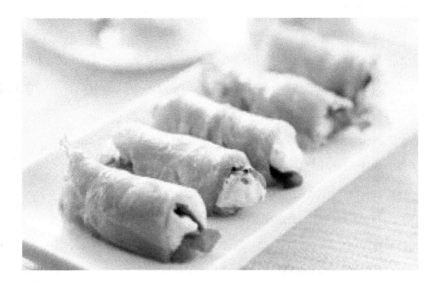

Preparation time: 10 minutes

Cooking time: 2 hours

Servings: 8

Ingredients:

- Smoked salmon – 4 strips, cut in half lengthways
- Firm cream cheese – ¼ lb., cut into 8 chunks
- Mozzarella cheese – ¼ lb., cut into 8 chunks
- Spring onion – 1, finely chopped
- Lemon – 1, zest
- Olive oil – 2 tbsp.

Directions:

1. Press one piece of mozzarella and one piece of cream cheese together. Sprinkle with a small amount of spring onion.
2. Wrap the cheese bundle in smoked salmon.
3. Repeat the process with the remaining Ingredients.
4. Drizzle oil into the Crock-Pot and place salmon bites in one layer into the pot.
5. Secure the lid and cook on low for 2 hours.
6. Garnish with lemon zest and serve.

Nutrition:

Calories: 195

Fat: 17.1g

Carbs: 3.7g

Protein: 7.9g

Smoked Lamb Chili

Preparation time: 10 minutes

Cooking time: 8 hours

Servings: 4

Ingredients

- 2 lbs. grass-fed ground lamb
- 8 bacon strips, diced
- 1 small onion, diced
- 3 tablespoons of chili powder
- 2 tablespoons of smoked paprika
- 4 teaspoons of cumin, ground
- 2 red bell pepper, seeded and diced
- Black pepper, to taste
- 4 garlic cloves, minced

Directions:

1. Start by putting all the **Ingredients** into your Slow cooker.
2. Cover its lid and cook for 8 hours on Medium settings.
3. Once done, remove its lid and mix well.
4. Garnish as desired.
5. Serve warm.

Nutrition:

Calories 511

Total Fat 18.5 g

Saturated Fat 11.5 g

Cholesterol 51 mg

Sodium 346 mg

Total Carbs 22 g

Sugar 0.5 g

Fiber 0.4 g

Potassium 123 mg

Protein 11.5 g

Lamb Chops Curry

Preparation time: 10 minutes

Cooking time: 6 hours

Servings: 2

Ingredients

- 1 lb. lamb loin chops
- 1 garlic clove, crushed
- ½ cup of bone broth
- 3/4 teaspoon of rosemary, dried, crushed
- 1 tablespoon of xanthan gum
- 1 ½ tablespoons of butter
- ½ small onion, sliced
- 3/4 cup of Sugar-free diced tomatoes
- 1 cup of carrots, peeled and sliced
- Salt and black pepper
- ½ tablespoon of cold water

Directions:

1. Start by putting all the **Ingredients** into your Slow cooker.
2. Cover its lid and cook for 6 hours on Low settings.
3. Once done, remove its lid and mix well.
4. Garnish as desired.
5. Serve warm.

Nutrition:

Calories 184

Total Fat 12.7 g

Saturated Fat 7.3 g

Cholesterol 35 mg

Sodium 222 mg

Total Carbs 6.3 g

Sugar 2.7 g

Fiber 1.6 g

Potassium 342mg

Protein 12.2 g

Dinner Lamb Shanks

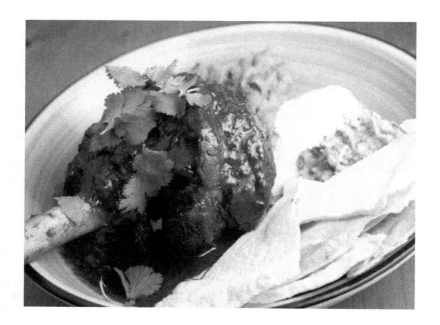

Preparation time: 10 minutes

Cooking time: 8 hours

Servings: 3

Ingredients

- 1 ½ lb. grass-fed lamb shanks, trimmed
- 1 tablespoon of olive oil
- 3/4 cup of bone broth
- ½ teaspoon of rosemary, dried, crushed
- 1 tablespoon of melted butter
- 3 whole garlic cloves, peeled
- Salt and black pepper, to taste

- 3/4 tablespoon of Sugar-free tomato paste
- 1 ¼ tablespoon of fresh lemon juice

Directions:

1. Start by putting all the **Ingredients** into your Slow cooker.
2. Cover its lid and cook for 8 hours on Low settings.
3. Once done, remove its lid and mix well.
4. Garnish as desired.
5. Serve warm.

Nutrition:

Calories 188

Total Fat 12.5 g

Saturated Fat 4.4 g

Cholesterol 53 mg

Sodium 1098 mg

Total Carbs 4.9 g

Sugar 0.3 g

Fiber 2 g

Potassium 332mg

Protein 14.6 g

Coconut Lamb Stew

Preparation time: 10 minutes

Cooking time: 10 hours

Servings: 2

Ingredients

- 1 lb. grass-fed lamb shoulder, cut into bite-sized pieces
- 1 tablespoon of curry powder, divided
- ¼ cup of unsweetened coconut milk
- 2 tablespoons of coconut cream
- 1 tablespoon of coconut oil
- 1 medium yellow onion, diced
- ½ cup of chicken broth
- 1 tablespoon of fresh lemon juice
- Salt and black pepper, to taste
- 2 tablespoons of fresh basil, diced

Directions:

1. Start by putting all the **Ingredients** into your Slow cooker except basil.
2. Cover its lid and cook for 10 hours on Low settings.
3. Once done, remove its lid and mix well.
4. Garnish with basil
5. Serve warm.

Nutrition:

Calories 141

Total Fat 11.3 g

Saturated Fat 3.8 g

Cholesterol 181 mg

Sodium 334 mg

Total Carbs 0.6 g

Sugar 0.5 g

Fiber 0 g

Potassium 332 mg

Protein 8.9 g

Herbed Lamb Stew

Preparation time: 10 minutes

Cooking time: 9 hours

Servings: 2

Ingredients

- 1 lb. grass-fed lamb shoulder, trimmed and cubed into 2-inch size
- 3/4 tablespoon of olive oil
- 1 celery stalk, diced
- 1 cup of tomatoes, diced
- 1 ½ tablespoon of fresh lemon juice
- ½ teaspoon of salt
- ½ teaspoon of black pepper
- ½ large green bell pepper, cut into 8 slices
- ½ large red bell pepper, cut into 8 slices
- ½ cup of bone broth
- ½ small onion, diced
- ½ tablespoon of garlic, minced
- ½ teaspoon of oregano, dried, crushed
- ½ teaspoon of dried basil, crushed

Directions:

1. Start by putting all the **Ingredients** into your Slow cooker.
2. Cover its lid and cook for 9 hours on Low settings.
3. Once done, remove its lid and mix well.

4. Garnish as desired.

5. Serve warm.

Nutrition:

Calories 260

Total Fat 22.9 g

Saturated Fat 7.3 g

Cholesterol 0 mg

Sodium 9 mg

Total Carbs 47 g

Sugar 1.8 g

Fiber 1.4 g

Protein 5.6 g

Vegetable Lamb Stew

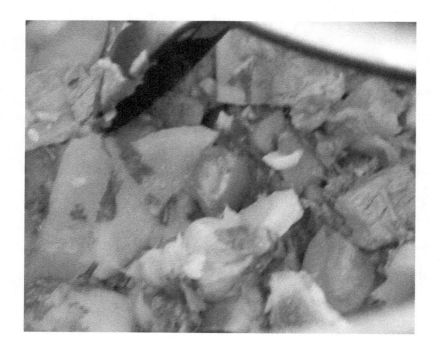

Preparation time: 10 minutes

Cooking time: 10.5 hours

Servings: 2

Ingredients

- 1 lb. cubed lamb stew meat
- 1 tablespoon of fresh ginger, grated
- ½ teaspoon of lime juice
- ¼ teaspoon of black pepper
- 3/4 cup of diced tomatoes
- ½ teaspoon of turmeric powder

- 1 ½ medium carrots, sliced
- 2 garlic cloves, minced
- ½ cup of coconut milk
- ¼ teaspoon of salt
- 1 tablespoon of olive oil
- ½ medium onion, diced
- ½ medium zucchini, diced

Directions:

1. Start by putting all the **Ingredients** into your Slow cooker except zucchini.
2. Cover its lid and cook for 10 hours on Low settings.
3. Once done, remove its lid and mix well.
4. Stir in zucchini and continue cooking for 30 minutes on high heat.
5. Garnish as desired.
6. Serve warm.

Nutrition:

Calories 108

Total Fat 9 g

Saturated Fat 4.3 g

Cholesterol 180 mg

Sodium 146 mg

Total Carbs 1.1 g

Sugar 0.5 g

Fiber 0.1 g

Protein 6 g

Lamb Leg with Thyme

Preparation time: 10 minutes

Cooking time: 10 hours

Servings: 4

Ingredients

- 2 lbs. leg of lamb
- 1 teaspoon of fine salt
- 2 ½ tablespoons of olive oil
- 6 sprigs thyme
- 1 ½ cup of bone broth
- 6 garlic cloves, minced
- 1 ½ teaspoon of black pepper
- 1 ½ small onion
- 3/4 cup of vegetable stock

Directions:

1. Start by putting all the **Ingredients** into your Slow cooker.
2. Cover its lid and cook for 10 hours on Low settings.
3. Once done, remove its lid and mix well.
4. Garnish as desired.
5. Serve warm.

Nutrition:

Calories 112

Total Fat 4.9 g

Saturated Fat 1.9 g

Cholesterol 10 mg

Sodium 355 mg

Total Carbs 1.9 g

Sugar 0.8 g

Fiber 0.4 g

Protein 3 g

Full Meal Turmeric Lamb

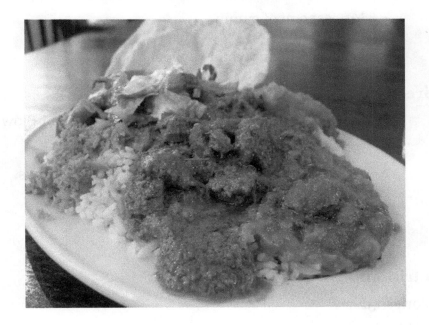

Preparation time: 10 minutes

Cooking time: 6 hours

Servings: 2

Ingredients

- ½ lb. ground lamb meat

- ½ cup of onion diced

- ½ tablespoon of garlic

- ½ tablespoon of minced ginger

- ¼ teaspoon of turmeric

- ¼ teaspoon of ground coriander

- ½ teaspoon of salt

- ¼ teaspoon of cumin

- ¼ teaspoon of cayenne pepper

Directions:

1. Start by putting all the **Ingredients** into your Slow cooker.
2. Cover its lid and cook for 6 hours on Low settings.
3. Once done, remove its lid and mix well.
4. Garnish as desired.
5. Serve warm.

Nutrition:

Calories 132

Total Fat 10.9 g

Saturated Fat 2.7 g

Cholesterol 164 mg

Sodium 65 mg

Total Carbs 3.3 g

Sugar 0.5 g

Fiber 2.3 g

Protein 6.3 g

Lamb Cauliflower Curry

Preparation time: 10 minutes

Cooking time: 10 hours.

Servings: 4

Ingredients

- 2 lbs. lamb roasted Wegmans

- 1 cup of onion soup

- ¼ cup of carrots

- 1 cup of cauliflower

- 1 cup of beef broth

Directions:

1. Start by putting all the **Ingredients** into your Slow cooker.
2. Cover its lid and cook for 10 hours on Low settings.
3. Once done, remove its lid and mix well.
4. Garnish as desired.
5. Serve warm.

Nutrition:

Calories 118

Total Fat 9.7 g

Saturated Fat 4.3 g

Cholesterol 228 mg

Sodium 160 mg

Total Carbs 0.5 g

Fiber 0 g

Sugar 0.5 g

Protein 7.4 g

Irish Chop Stew

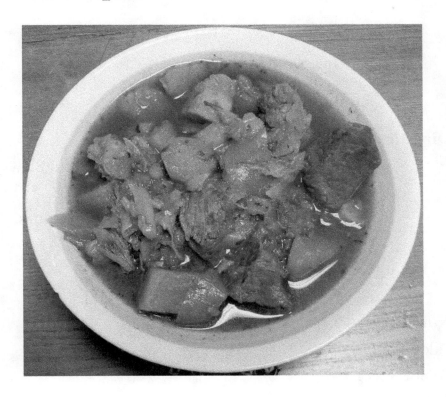

Preparation time: 10 minutes

Cooking time: 10 hours

Servings: 8

Ingredients

- 8 lamb shoulder chops, cubed

- 8 large onions, sliced into thin rounds

- 4 cups of water

- 4 tablespoons of olive oil

- 9 large carrots, chunked

- 4 sprigs thyme

- 2 teaspoons of salt

- 2 teaspoons of black pepper

Directions:

1. Start by putting all the **Ingredients** into your Slow cooker.
2. Cover its lid and cook for 10 hours on Low settings.
3. Once done, remove its lid and mix well.
4. Garnish as desired.
5. Serve warm.

Nutrition:

Calories 280

Total Fat 23 g

Saturated Fat 13.8 g

Cholesterol 82 mg

Sodium 28 mg

Total Carbs 3.1 g

Fiber 2.5 g

Sugar 0.5 g

Protein 3.9 g

Picante Glazed Chops

Preparation time: 10 minutes

Cooking time: 6 hours

Servings: 6

Ingredients

- 6 lamb chops, bone-in
- 1 ¼ cup of Picante sauce
- 1 cup of cherry tomatoes
- 3 tablespoons of olive oil
- 3 tablespoons of almond flour
- 3 tablespoons of brown swerve, packed

Directions:

1. Start by putting all the **Ingredients** into your Slow cooker.
2. Cover its lid and cook for 6 hours on Low settings.
3. Once done, remove its lid and mix well.
4. Garnish as desired.
5. Serve warm.

Nutrition:

Calories 206

Total Fat 20.8 g

Saturated Fat 14.2 g

Cholesterol 315 mg

Sodium 35 mg

Total Carbs 2.6 g

Fiber 0.1 g

Sugar 1.5 g

Protein 4.2 g

Pomegranate Lamb

Preparation time: 10 minutes

Cooking time: 10 hours 15 minutes

Servings: 4

Ingredients

- 1 leg of lamb, boneless (tied)
- 1 cup of pomegranate juice
- 1 cup of white wine
- 1 cup of chicken stock
- ½ cup of pomegranate seeds
- 4 mint leaves
- 4 cloves garlic, peeled and minced
- 1 teaspoon of black pepper, ground
- 1 teaspoon of salt
- 3 tablespoons of olive oil

Directions:

1. Start by throwing all the Ingredients except the pomegranate seeds, butter, and flour into your Slow cooker.
2. Cover its lid and cook for 10 hours on Low settings.
3. Once done, remove its lid and mix well.
4. Slice the slow-cooked lamb then transfer to a plate
5. Mix flour with butter in a small bowl then pour into the slow cooker.

6. Continue cooking the remaining sauce for 15 minutes on high heat.

7. Pour this sauce around the slices lamb.

8. Garnish with pomegranate seeds.

9. Serve warm.

Nutrition:

Calories 225

Total Fat 20.4 g

Saturated Fat 8.7 g

Cholesterol 30 mg

Sodium 135 mg

Total Carbs 7.7 g

Fiber 4.3 g

Sugar 2.2 g

Protein 5.2 g

Persian Lamb Curry

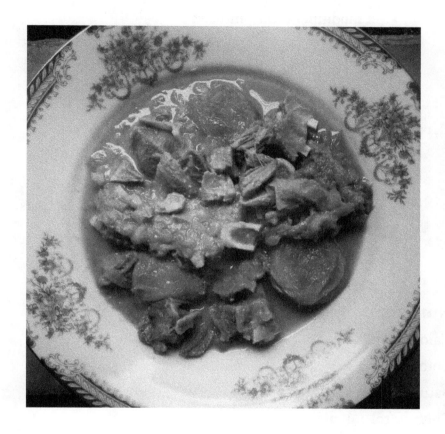

Preparation time: 10 minutes

Cooking time: 10 hours

Servings: 6

Ingredients

- 1 tablespoon of turmeric
- 2 teaspoons of black pepper
- 1 teaspoon of salt

- 1 teaspoon of crushed red pepper flakes
- 3 tablespoons of extra virgin olive oil
- 2 medium onions, minced
- 3 lbs. lamb meat, cut into chunks
- 3 tablespoons of tomato paste
- ¼ cup of cilantro, diced

Directions:

1. Start by putting all the Ingredients into your Slow cooker except cilantro.
2. Cover its lid and cook for 10 hours on Low settings.
3. Once done, remove its lid and mix well.
4. Garnish with cilantro.
5. Serve warm.

Nutrition:

Calories 376

Total Fat 12.1 g

Saturated Fat 14.2 g

Cholesterol 195 mg

Sodium 73 mg

Total Carbs 4.6 g

Fiber 3.1 g

Sugar 2.1 g

Protein 25.7 g

Indian Lamb Stew

Preparation time: 10 minutes
Cooking time: 10 hours 15 minutes
Servings: 8
Ingredients

- 2 tablespoons of sweet paprika
- 1 ½ teaspoons of cayenne pepper
- 1 cup of Greek yogurt
- ¼ cup of vegetable oil
- 4 lbs. boneless lamb shoulder
- 1 ½ teaspoons of ground ginger
- 1 ½ teaspoon of ground coriander
- ½ teaspoon of ground turmeric
- ¼ teaspoon of cloves, ground
- 2 small cinnamon sticks
- 8 cardamom pods
- 1 medium tomato, diced
- Black pepper
- 1 tablespoon of xanthan gum
- 2 tablespoons of water

Directions:

1. Start by throwing all the **Ingredients** except the butter and flour into your Slow cooker.
2. Cover its lid and cook for 10 hours on Low settings.
3. Once done, remove its lid and mix well.

4. Mix corn starch and water in a small bowl then pour into the slow cooker.
5. Continue cooking the remaining sauce for 15 minutes on high heat until it thickens.
6. Garnish as desired.
7. Serve warm.

Nutrition:

Calories 265

Total Fat 26.1 g

Saturated Fat 7.8 g

Cholesterol 143 mg

Sodium 65 mg

Total Carbs 5.9 g

Fiber 3.2 g

Sugar 1.3 g

Protein 6.1 g